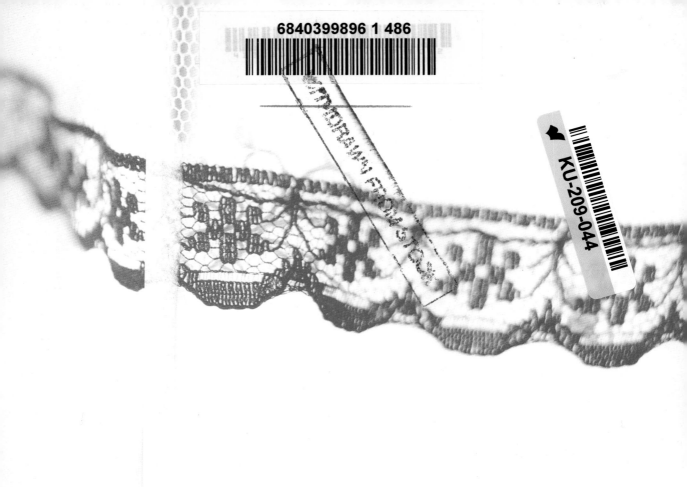

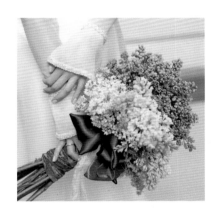

HOW TO BE A

beautiful
bride

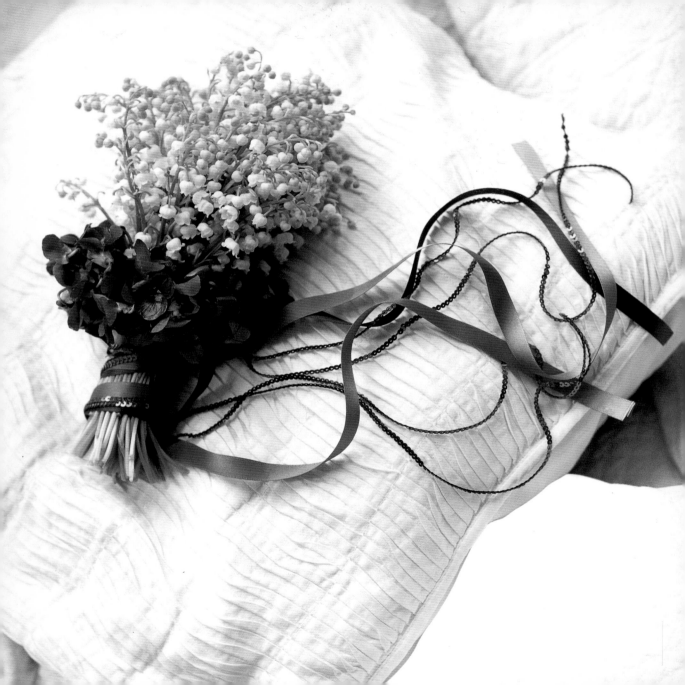

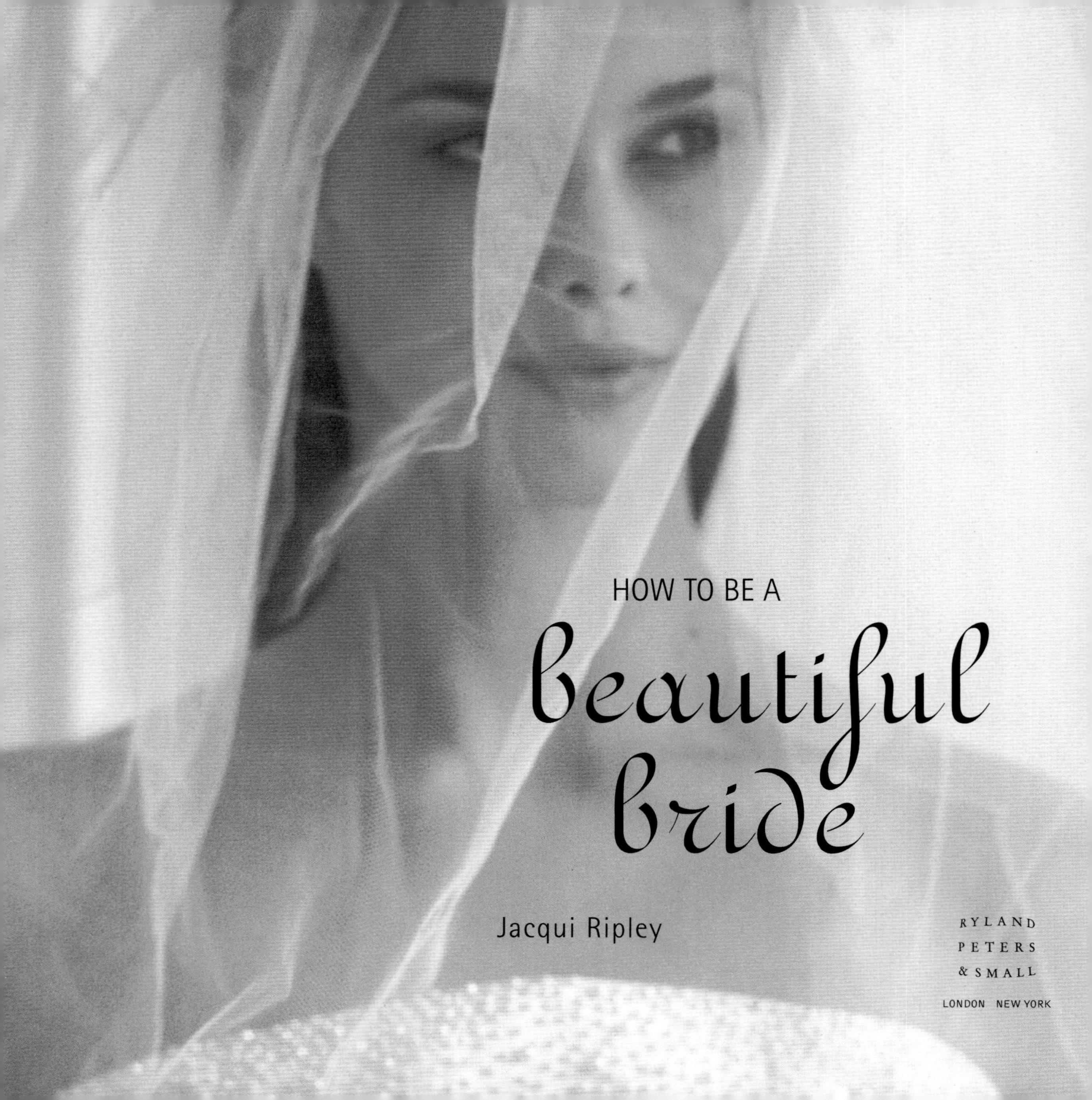

HOW TO BE A

beautiful
bride

Jacqui Ripley

RYLAND
PETERS
& SMALL

LONDON   NEW YORK

SENIOR DESIGNERS Sonya Nathoo and Sally Powell
COMMISSIONING EDITOR Annabel Morgan
LOCATION RESEARCH Tracy Ogino
PRODUCTION Gemma Moules
ART DIRECTOR Anne-Marie Bulat
PUBLISHING DIRECTOR Alison Starling

First published in Great Britain in 2007
by Ryland Peters & Small
20–21 Jockey's Fields
London WC1R 4BW
www.rylandpeters.com
10 9 8 7 6 5 4 3 2 1

Text copyright © Jacqui Ripley 2007
Design and photography copyright
© Ryland Peters & Small 2007

ISBN-10: 1-84597-331-3
ISBN-13: 978-1-84597-331-5

A CIP record is available from the British
Library.

Printed in China.

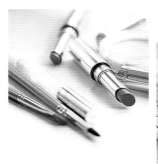
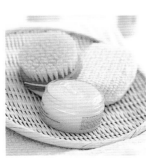

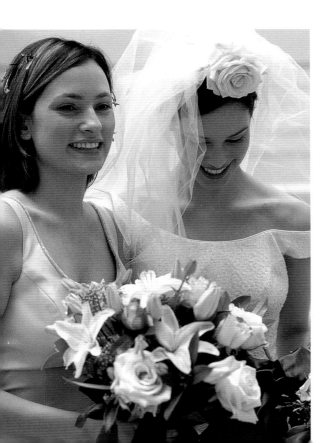

contents

introduction

Planning a wedding is fun, exciting and stressful all at the same time. But the most important factor for the bride is making sure she steals the limelight on her big day. Every bride wants to treasure magical memories of her wedding day forever, and for her look to be timeless. Finding your dream dress, planning your hair and make-up, getting started on figure-fixing exercises, and choosing accessories, are all at the forefront of a bride's mind.

If you're stressing over all these details, then relax. Within these pages is a multitude of inspired ideas you'll love, along with expert tips to ensure you will look and feel beautiful and to help you radiate an aura of serenity and happiness on your big day.

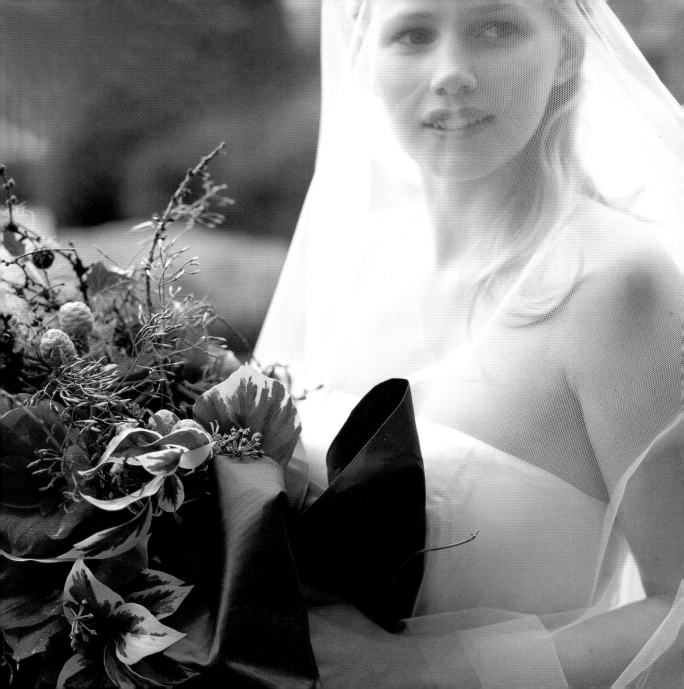

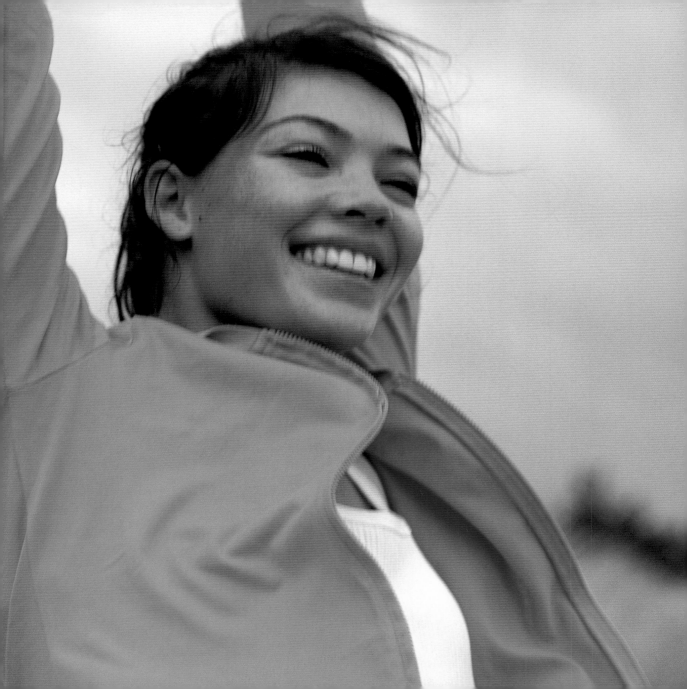

getting in shape

Being tight, toned and flab-free isn't as hard
as you think. The trick to looking fabulous in
your wedding gown is to tackle any problem
areas by using troubleshooting exercises that
will shape and define your figure.

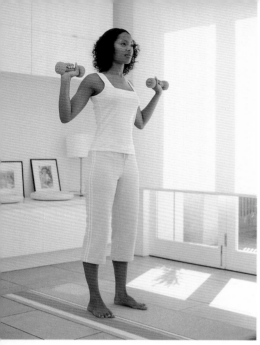

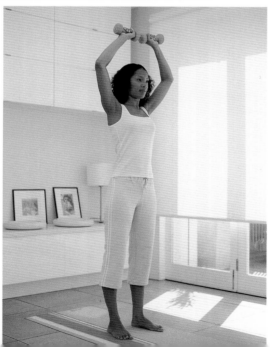

shoulders and bust

Hitting the gym to get fit and firm alongside organising one of the biggest days of your life can seem too much to take on. But focusing on improving your problem areas will keep your fitness plan realistic and achievable.

SHOULDER TONER

This exercise gives your shoulders definition – ideal if your dress is strappy or strapless. It's easy to overlook shoulders, but by defining them you keep your arms looking shapelier too.

1 Stand with your feet shoulder-width apart, tummy pulled in and shoulders back and down. Hold a 2–3 kg dumbbell in each hand with palms facing outwards. Keep arms bent at 90 degrees and weights held at shoulder level.

2 Press dumbbells straight upwards, raising your arms overhead. Keep arms as close to your ears as possible while raising your arms into an arch.

3 Lower the weights to the starting position. Rest for a moment, then repeat the exercise. Start with one set of 10, increasing to three sets of 15.

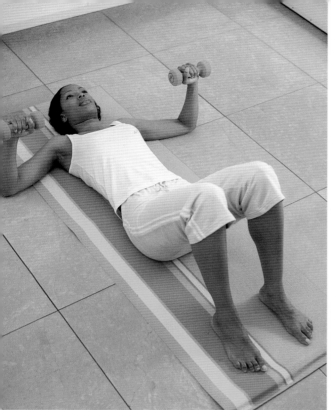
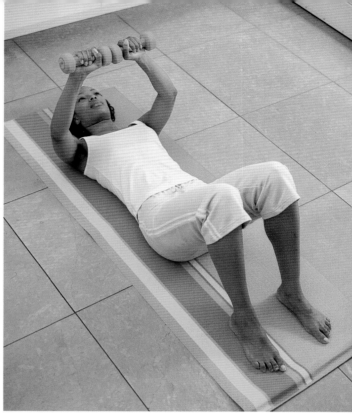

BUST FIRMER

Unfortunately exercises cannot alter the size of your bust, but they can strengthen and tone the surrounding pectoral muscles (the underlying muscles around the breasts) for a better uplift.

1 Lie back on the floor with knees bent, holding a dumbbell in each hand. Keep elbows bent at 90 degrees and the upper arms resting on the floor.

2 Slowly press hands straight up and bring weights together over your chest – not your head. Lower arms back down to the starting position. Rest and repeat. Start with one set of 10, increasing to three sets of 15.

• Palm presses are a great no-fuss bust-boosting exercise. Press your palms together under your chin and in front of your bust, as if praying. Hold for a few seconds, relax, and then repeat 20 times.

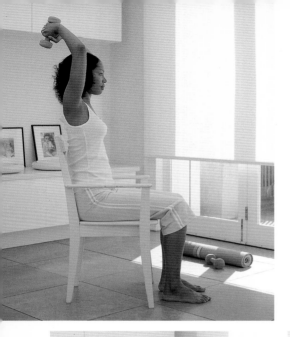

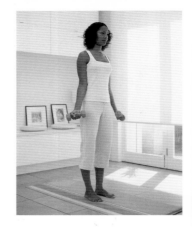

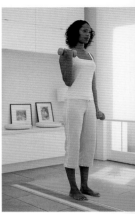

arm shapers

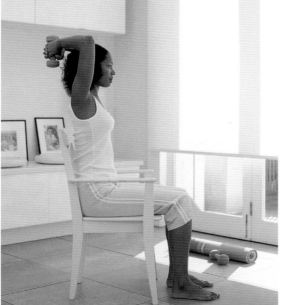

For toned, taut arms, your triceps and biceps (as well as the upper back) need to be addressed. The secret is to conjure up a mental image of yourself in a sleeveless top – that should send you running for the dumbbells!

FOR THE TRICEPS (LEFT)

1 Sit on a chair, with head up, back straight and feet on the floor. Hold one dumbbell vertical to the floor with both hands overhead.

2 Keeping your upper arms in place, slowly lower the dumbbell straight down behind your head as low as you can comfortably go, keeping elbows at one fixed point.

3 Raise the dumbbell back up over your head until arms are fully extended. Start with one set of 10, slowly increasing to three sets of 15.

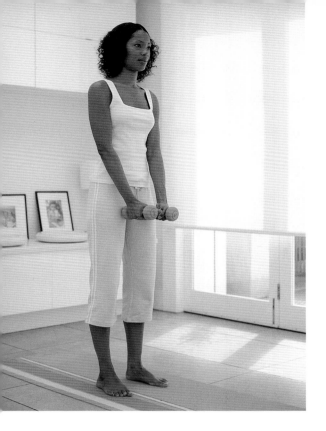
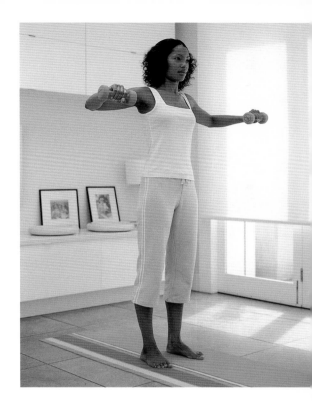

FOR THE BICEPS (ABOVE LEFT)

1 Stand with feet shoulder-width apart and arms by your sides, holding a dumbbell in each hand.

2 Leaving your left arm relaxed and pointing towards the floor, slowly bend your right arm up to a 45-degree angle and continue to bring the weight right up to your shoulder. Lower until the arm is straight.

3 Repeat with the opposite arm. Aim for three sets of 10–15 repetitions per arm.

FOR THE UPPER BACK (ABOVE)

1 Stand with feet hip-width apart and a dumbbell in each hand, palms facing inwards and arms in front of the body. Keep elbows relaxed and tummy pulled in.

2 Slowly lift your arms out to the side, keeping elbows relaxed. Your elbows should be bent at 90 degrees and parallel to the floor. Raise your arms no higher than shoulder level. Hold for a couple of seconds, then lower. Start with one set of 10, increasing to three sets of 15.

waist and stomach

WAISTING AWAY

A defined waist gives any figure better proportion. Work your waist muscles diligently, and you will transform your figure from shapeless to hourglass.

WAIST STRENGTHENER (BELOW)

1 Lie on your side and place your elbow under your shoulder so it acts as a support. Place one foot on top of the other and pull in your tummy muscles.
2 Slowly raise yourself up, using your obliques (waist muscles) to keep the position. Lift your arm over and above your head. Hold for a count of 10–20 seconds. Repeat on the other side.

TWIST CRUNCHES

Lie with knees bent and feet flat on the ground. Place your hands under your head with elbows out to the side. Keeping hips still, slowly rotate the upper body to your right, so the upper back and shoulders come off the floor. Lower, and repeat on the other side.

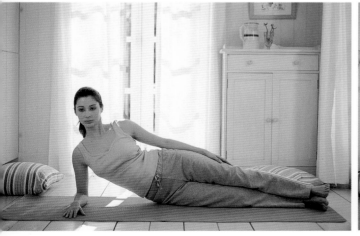
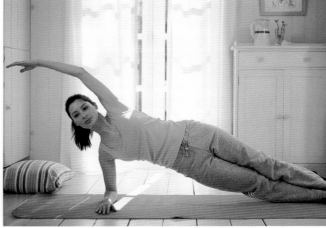

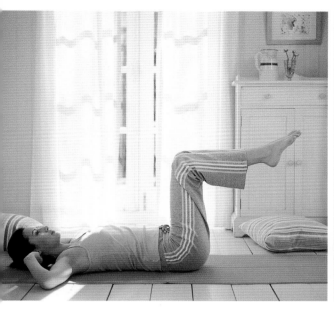
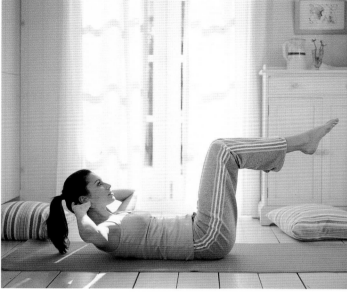

STOMACH SMOOTHERS

A flatter stomach gives you added confidence, and helps to support your back and improve your posture.

MID-AB CRUNCH (ABOVE)

1 Lie flat on your back with arms at your sides and legs raised in the air at a 90-degree angle to your body.
2 Push your lower back firmly into the floor and raise your upper body with your hands behind your head, crunching upwards. Do two sets of 30 repetitions.

LOWER-AB CRUNCH (RIGHT)

1 Lie on your back with hands under your bottom. This will tilt the pelvis up slightly and support the lower back.
2 Lift your legs up and bend your knees almost to a 90-degree angle. Lift your pelvis and buttocks back towards your ribcage. Aim for two sets of 30 repetitions.

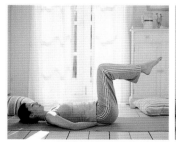
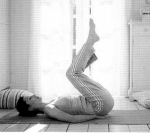

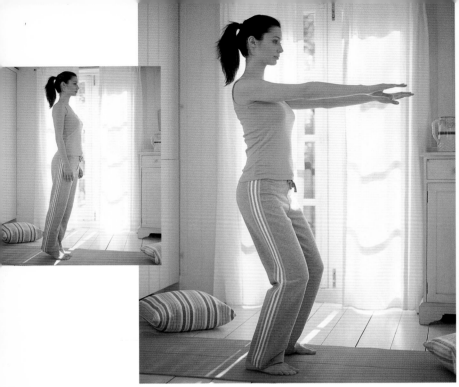
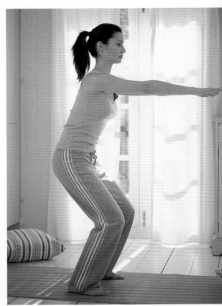

bottoms and legs

THIGH AND BOTTOM BOOSTERS
Exercise can help bottoms and thighs tone up quickly, blessing you with a more streamlined shape.

SQUATS (ABOVE)
1 Stand with feet shoulder-width apart, toes turned out and knees slightly bent.

2 Slowly lower yourself into a squat (as if sitting down) until your knees are directly above your ankles. Return to starting position. Repeat 15 times for three sets.

BUTTOCK CLENCHES
When sitting or queuing, squeeze and clench your buttocks for five seconds, then release. Repeat 20 times.

THIGH TRIMMER (BELOW)

1 Lie on your right side, with head, shoulders and hips aligned. Support your head with your right hand and place your left arm in front of you for stability. Bend your left leg and place it in front of your right leg.

2 Keeping your right leg straight and foot flexed, slowly raise your right leg about 15–20 cm off the ground. Hold your leg for a second at the top of the movement, then lower. Repeat for 8–12 reps for three sets. Repeat on the other side.

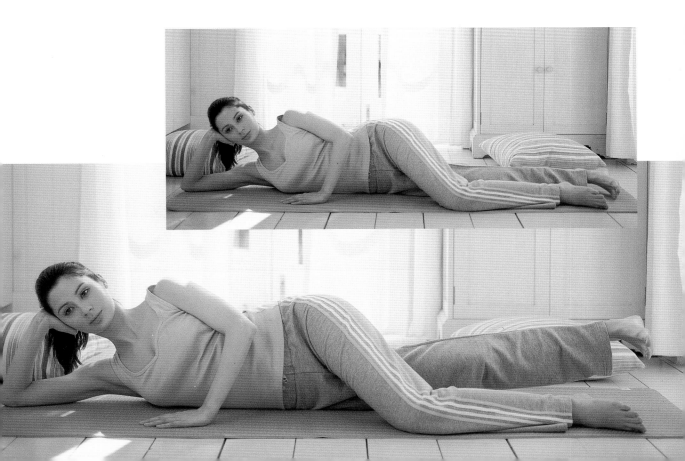

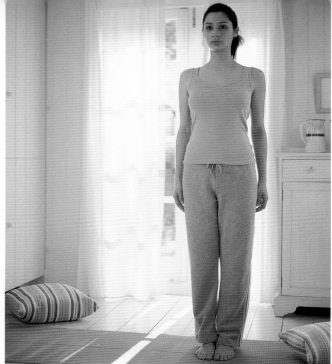
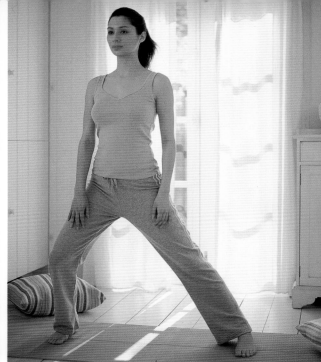

LEG SLIMMER (ABOVE)

Our legs are exercised each day through walking, but you can slot in a few specific moves if you want to tone your legs faster.

1 Stand tall, feet together, toes facing forwards. Take a wide step to the right with your right foot and bend your right knee, so you're in a side lunge.

2 Place your hands just above your right knee, hold for one, then squeeze your bottom and return to the starting position. Hold for one, then lunge again. Repeat for 15 reps on each side for three sets.

CALF SHAPER

1 Stand with feet together, toes facing forward and arms by your sides. Lift your heels and roll onto the balls of the feet. Hold for a second, then lower. Repeat 20 times.

WALL SQUATS

Stand 60cm away from a wall with arms by your sides. Sit back, as if onto a chair, until your back is flat against the wall and your thighs are parallel to the floor. Hold this position until your legs become fatigued, then lower yourself to the floor. Repeat up to 10 times.

a class act to follow

To help take your figure from average to amazing, why not try a class to stretch, tone and burn off calories?

PILATES A slow and precise form of exercise which helps gain body awareness. Helps lengthen and strengthen muscles, as well as improving posture and rebalancing the body.

YOGA Ancient healing systems of exercise that can improve energy, increase flexibility, build strength, centre your emotions and induce a sense of calm. Start off with relaxing Hatha yoga or, if you fancy something more challenging, try the aerobic-style Ashtanga.

AEROBICS A fantastic way to get fit while having fun. Covers all the body bases, from stretching through to conditioning and cardiovascular work.

BELLY DANCING Lots of fun, as well as a great workout for the midriff. The deep abdominal muscles and pelvic floor are worked, and belly dancing also shapes and sculpts the waist, hips and thighs.

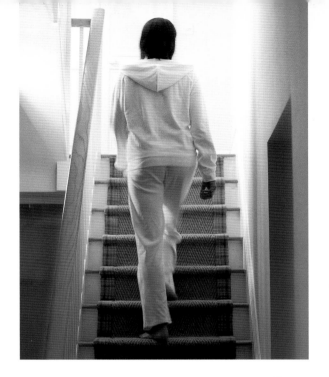

EASY MOVES

☆ *Take the stairs for an all-over bottom and leg shaper. Take two at a time for better results.*

☆ *Throw on some tunes and dance. Your body will thank you for it.*

☆ *Walk in heels. It trains your legs to produce muscle, especially in the calves and thighs.*

☆ *Focus on pulling your abs back towards your spine at all times. You'll target the deep abdominal muscles that are responsible for keeping your tummy taut.*

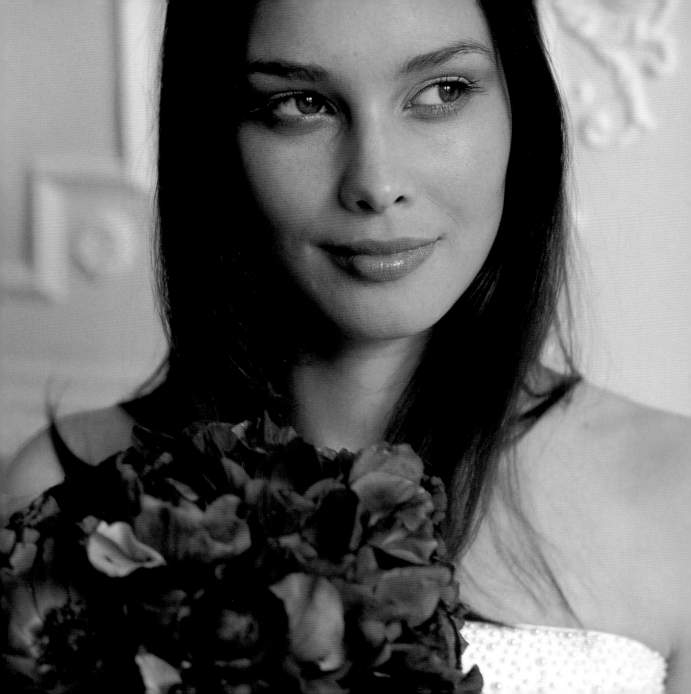

getting gorgeous

Great skin, strong nails, glossy hair – ever thought there might be a connection? Good nutrition is the foundation for all these things, and eating the right foods is one of the hardest-working beauty treatments.

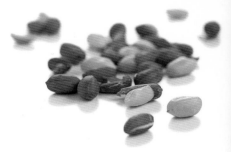

becoming a beauty gourmet

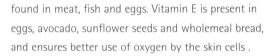

'ACE IT' Super skin relies on vitamins A, C and E, otherwise known as antioxidants. They protect skin from free-radical damage. Beta-carotene is found in brightly coloured vegetables and fruits and is converted by the body into vitamin A, which prevents dry skin. Vitamin C plays a leading role in the production of collagen and is found in meat, fish and eggs. Vitamin E is present in eggs, avocado, sunflower seeds and wholemeal bread, and ensures better use of oxygen by the skin cells .

EAT FISH A couple of portions of oily fish a week will help keep hair nourished and glossy and nails strong. Sardines, salmon and mackerel all contain omega-3 fatty acids, which are essential for beauty maintenance.

ZOOM IN ON ZINC Top up your zinc levels, as skin, nails and hair feed off this nutrient. Find it in nuts, seeds, wheatgerm and poultry.

PACK IN PROTEIN Hair is a protein, nails are made up of layers of a protein called keratin, and skin cells cannot repair themselves without sufficient amounts. Amino acids are the building blocks of protein, and are found in meat, poultry, fish, eggs, nuts, pulses and beans.

DETOXIFYING DRINKS Sip dandelion tea to help decongest the kidneys and liver. Drink a cup three times a day to help your body get rid of waste products and detox stressed skin.

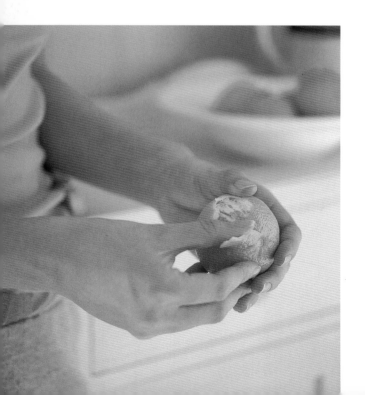

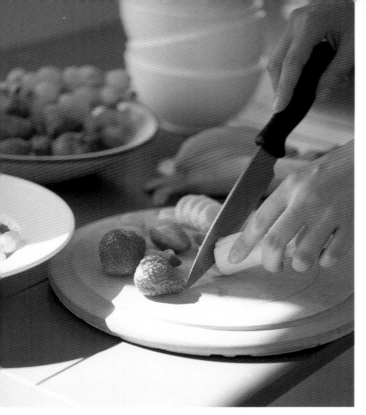

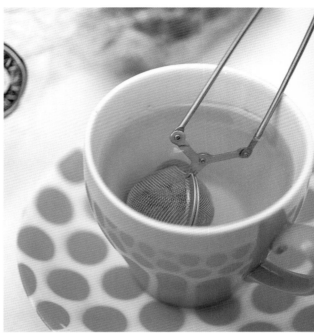

ENERGY FOODS TO GO Use food as an energizer to put sparkle into your skin and eyes.
• Pick the right fruit. Apples, pears and berries are all slow-releasing fruits and therefore provide more sustained energy.
• Fill yourself with beans. Baked beans, kidney beans, chickpeas and lentils are top energy foods.
• Avoid fast foods. Too many processed foods make skin sluggish and hair listless. Eat foods that are as fresh as possible.

SUPPLEMENT SMART
A varied diet should address all your nutritional and beauty needs, but the following minerals are commonly depleted in women:
☆ *Magnesium. Helps to repair and maintain body cells. Important for strong teeth. RDA 300mg.*
☆ *Iron. A deficiency shows in brittle fingernails, hair loss and tiredness. RDA 14mg.*
☆ *Zinc. Essential for cell repair. RDA 15mg.*

skin spoilers

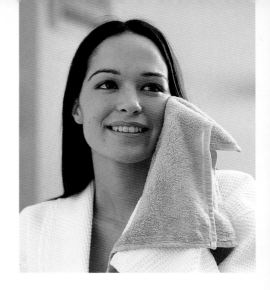

Falling into bad lifestyle habits can affect the way your skin looks and behaves. Experts now believe that changing your attitude towards the following can really benefit the overall appearance of your skin.

TOO MUCH ALCOHOL Alcohol constricts the blood vessels and dehydrates the skin, giving it a ruddy, weatherbeaten look. Alcohol robs your skins of essential vitamins and nutrients and impairs the cleansing ability of the liver. If the liver isn't flushing out toxins adequately, the skin will start to look sallow.

TOO LITTLE WATER The difference between the look of a grape and a raisin is water! Insufficient water intake can quickly result in a spotty and lacklustre complexion. Did you know that one caffeinated drink takes four glasses of moisture from your body? Drink 8–10 glasses a day, and carry a water bottle around with you.

SMOKING You don't even have to be a smoker for your skin to suffer from this nasty habit. A passive smoker's skin is at risk, too. Apart from the increased likelihood of premature ageing, smoking starves the skin of oxygen and reduces its ability to generate collagen. Nicotine also deprives the skin of essential nutrients; namely, vitamins A and C.

YO-YO DIETING An endless cycle of constant weight gain and loss stretches the skin to the point of no return, and this is where elasticity drops significantly. A healthy vanity drop would be up to 1kg a week – any more than that and you will be losing lean muscle tissue, which is when the face can start to look gaunt.

EXCESS SUGAR Our sugar intake has risen alarmingly. When there's too much sugar in your bloodstream, the excess sticks to protein fibres between your skin cells, causing premature ageing and degeneration. To beat sugar cravings, make sure you eat little and often, and combine protein-rich foods with carbohydrates.

FOODS THAT BEAUTIFY

☆ *Avocado. A skin treat rich in vitamin E, which is essential for the health of the eyes.*

☆ *Beetroot. A rich source of iron, vitamin A, vitamin C and calcium. Also contains other nutrients that are excellent for skin and strengthening blood vessels.*

☆ *Blueberries. A superfood with blood-cleansing properties. A good source of vitamins and minerals.*

☆ *Grapes. Boast polyphenols – power antioxidants. Have a 'grape day' and you'll rest your digestion, speed up the detox process and help your skin.*

☆ *Carrots. A good all-rounder, high in fibre, vitamin C and beta-carotene.*

☆ *Lemons. A great cleanser, with precious bioflavonoids and twice as much vitamin C as oranges. Slice into hot water and sip instead of tea or coffee.*

skin fitness

For a flawless complexion, it's essential to adopt a good skin fitness regime in the run-up to your wedding day. Opt for a daily routine of facial exercises and massage, along with an efficient care and cleansing regime.

FACIAL WORKOUTS Holistic facialists believe facial exercises give a natural facelift and restore radiance. While facials will unblock pores, it's the supportive facial muscles that keep skin firm. Exercises help in achieving this as well as delivering improved collagen production — the inner mattress of the skin.

JAW FIRMER Sit upright and tilt your head back towards the ceiling. Keeping your lips closed, start a chewing motion. You will feel the muscles working in your neck and jaw area. Repeat 20 times.

EYE TONER Press two fingers on each side of your head at the temples, while opening and closing your eyes quickly. Repeat up to 10 times.

FOREHEAD SMOOTHER Draw your eyebrows down over your eyes. Wrinkle your nose up as far as possible. Hold for a count of 10, relax, and repeat five times.

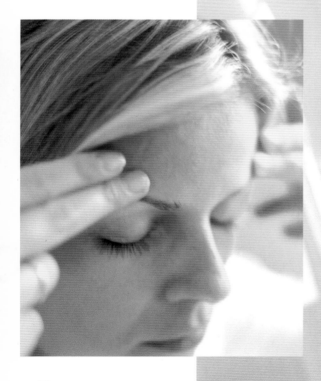

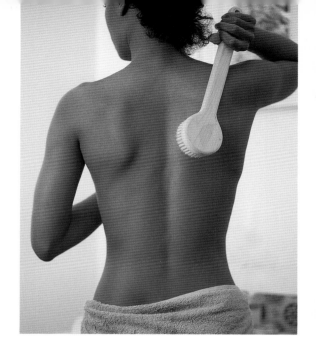

FEEL-GOOD MASSAGE Massage stimulates blood flow, drains toxins and relaxes. Face tapping is a good place to start. Make light, quick taps with the pads of your middle fingers all over your face. Use your palms and take sweeping upward movements over your face using a favourite moisturiser.

SKIN STRATEGIES Lay down skin commandments in your quest for gorgeous skin. Cleansing, moisturising and exfoliating are fundamental should-dos. Skin problems arise when dirt and dead skin cells aren't swiftly dealt with. Good skin relies on moisturising, which swells skin cells, leaving skin plump and healthy.

ALL AGLOW Exfoliation illuminates your complexion. A twice-weekly scrub will help control breakouts, alleviate dryness and minimise the appearance of fine lines. Two ingredients that have been scientifically proven to bless skin with radiance are alpha-hydroxyl acids and retinols. Look for them in moisturisers and night creams.

A SPOT OF BOTHER? High levels of the stress hormone cortisol and adrenaline cause acne. Do not hope it will clear up by itself – see your doctor to ask about antibiotics months before your wedding. Use non-comedogenic products and look for products containing salicylic acid, which unclogs pores and gets rid of dead skin cells.

SKIN TIPS

☆ *Energize eyes by tapping on a light eye cream with your ring finger before bed.*

☆ *Use a mask while bathing. Steam opens pores and encourages deeper penetration.*

☆ *Sun damage is the top reason skin turns dingy. Wear moisturizer with an SPF and fake your glow.*

☆ *For on-the-day blemishes, wrap an ice cube in muslin and press onto the spot. This will instantly take down swelling, making it easy to cover.*

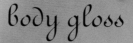

body gloss

For a smoother, sleeker body, capture some all-over skin radiance with these brilliant bare-it-all tips.

GLEAM ON An all-over scrub will remove dead cells from the skin's surface, leaving it soft and more receptive to moisture. Body brush from the feet upwards before showering, or use a scrub. Pay attention to less obvious areas, such as ankles, knees, elbows and the back of arms when using a scrub. These are places where dead cells build up, leaving skin thickened and dull. If you find the back awkward to reach, use a towel. Hold one end over your shoulder and the other down by your opposite hip, then slowly rub back and forth slowly. Switch sides to make sure you've exfoliated your entire back.

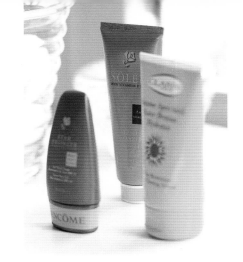

MUST-HAVE MOISTURE Adequate moisture will leave skin looking supple, with a more even skintone. When using body products, remember the product needs to work at a deeper level, so it takes longer for results to become apparent. Start slathering on the body cream early for visible results on your wedding day. For maximum moisturising, don't apply straight after bathing. Wait until your skin is completely dry; otherwise it ends up absorbing moisture too quickly.

THE BUZZ ON FUZZ Hair removal is a non-negotiable beauty chore. Stubbly or hairy underarms and legs don't make for a great photo opportunity! Hair removal should be done before applying fake tan – tanning lotion can get caught up around short hairs and give a spotty finish. Shaving is fast; just make sure your blade is new, and use shaving foam to prevent any nicks. Waxing and cream depilatories make for a satiny smooth finish (wax at least two days before your wedding to allow skin to settle). Prevent any ingrowing hairs by exfoliating the legs and applying tea tree cream.

HONEY-KISSED SKIN A fake tan warms up skin, evens out imperfections and makes you look slimmer. Pulling off a credible colour is all in the application. Apply the tan two nights before the wedding, to avoid stains on your dress and to allow the colour to develop fully. First exfoliate, dry and moisturise the body. Start at your feet and work upwards, applying self-tan on one section of your body at a time. Smooth over skin with long, vertical strokes, followed by horizontal ones, until the cream is completely absorbed. Use less cream on your joints, where colour can collect in creases. Use a separate product for the face and apply from the centre of the face outwards. Blend at the jawline and around the ears. Keep cream away from the hairline and eyebrows.

getting hair happy

Most brides have an idea of how they want their hair to look on their wedding day, but you also need to think about the overall condition, cut and colour of your hair.

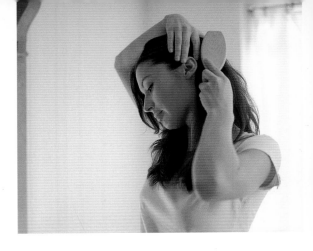

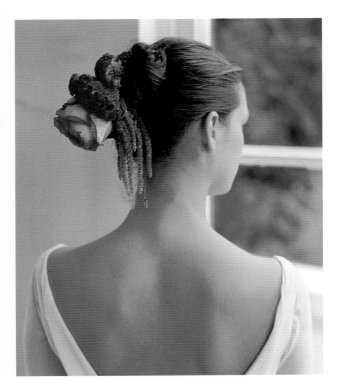

HIGH-CLASS HAIR Washing your hair is the single most important aspect of hair health. Shampooing stimulates the hair follicles, and hair should look its best when it is freshly washed. If it doesn't, you're either using the wrong products or not shampooing correctly. For a foolproof technique, apply shampoo, gently knead the scalp for about a minute, then rinse thoroughly.

CLEVER CONDITIONING Follow shampoo with the correct conditioner for your hair type. Pay particular attention to the ends – they're always drier. If hair feels rough, look to creamier formulations or invest in an intensive conditioning mask.

A CUT ABOVE THE REST Good-hair days start with a great cut. Visit your hairdresser at least six months before the big day for a chat. If you need to grow out a fringe or old colour, this should give you enough time. It's also the right time to experiment with new styles.

If you're thinking of changing your style, bring a picture of what you want along with you. A picture is worth a thousand words! If your hair has been damaged by chemicals or over-processing, the results will be split ends. The only cure is to snip them off. A centimetre off the ends every six weeks will result in healthier hair.

TUNE INTO COLOUR Great colour freshens up your hairstyle, injects volume and bumps up shine. Get your hair coloured at least two weeks before your wedding, to give it time to readjust. A good colourist will give their client plenty of advice before going for a colour switch. From subtle highlights to a full-on transformation, you need to take into account your skintone.

COLOUR TIPS
• Warm up pale skin with honey blonde, reddish gold or warm brown tones.
• Olive-skinned beauties should opt for auburn, amber and caramel shades. Avoid anything bleached or brassy.
• If you have yellow skin, keep your base colour dark, and highlight with lighter toffee browns. Anything too blonde will wash you out.
• Dark brown skin suits deep browns like mahogany and chestnut, which give hair richness and depth.

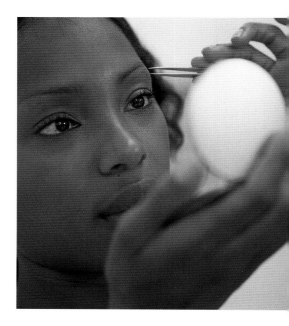

...DON'T FORGET EYEBROWS
☆ *Eyebrows frame your face, and playing around with your hair colour can alter the balance of your features.*
☆ *Only tint your eyebrows darker if you have chosen a darker hair colour.*
☆ *If going a lot lighter than your natural hair colour, brows should be lightened slightly.*
☆ *You can use a cream bleach to lighten eyebrows or an eyelash dyeing kit to darken them, but unless you really know what you're doing it's a job best left to the beauty experts!*

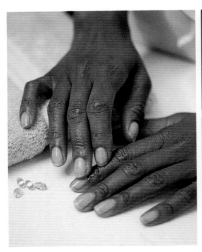
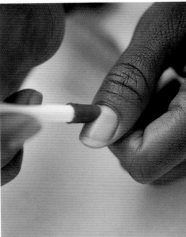
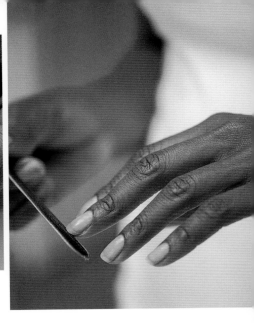

Details that make a difference

When it comes to understated but elegant bridal style, grooming is the watchword. Subtle touches to hands, nails and feet will bring a look together.

HANDS-ON BEAUTY

Holding the bouquet, signing the register and admiring the ring makes a bride's hands really important on the big day. You want hands to look great, so start wearing rubber gloves when washing up and doing household chores. Like your face, give hands a 'facial' by exfoliating and moisturising regularly. When applying a face mask, put some on the backs of the hands as well.

PRETTY AND POLISHED

If you're a chronic nail biter, start booking a professional weekly manicure or doing your own. It gets you into the habit of having groomed nails. Another tip is to wear brightly coloured nail polish. When your nails get near your mouth, the colour will grab your attention and hopefully you will stop nibbling! To keep your nails looking slick, file them into a squoval shape (neither square nor round). Don't pick things up with your nails – use the pads of your fingers instead. When it comes to choosing polish, stick to sophisticated shades such as nude, beige or pale pink.

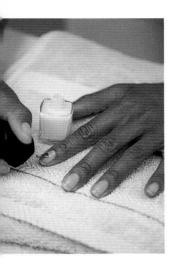

CUTE CUTICLES

For polish to look good, your cuticles need to be in excellent shape. Get into the habit of applying a cuticle oil around your cuticles before bed every night. This ensures dry skin won't ruin the look of your manicure. For an instant improvement in the condition of your nails, break open a vitamin E capsule and massage the oil into the cuticles. Massaging the nail plate with the base of your thumb brings the blood to the surface, which stimulates growth.

THE FOOTSIE LOW-DOWN

Even if you're not wearing open-toed shoes, bridal feet should still be buffed and polished. The skin on the foot is unique, as it's four times thicker than anywhere else on the body. Calluses are a common problem – get rid of these hard areas of dry skin by buffing the heels and sides of the foot with a pumice stone twice a week. Always dry feet properly; moist areas are a breeding ground for fungal infections. Apply foot cream and cuticle oil last thing at night to give the moisture a chance to soak in.

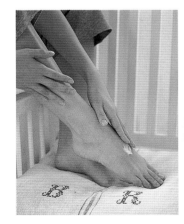

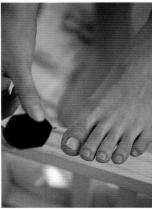

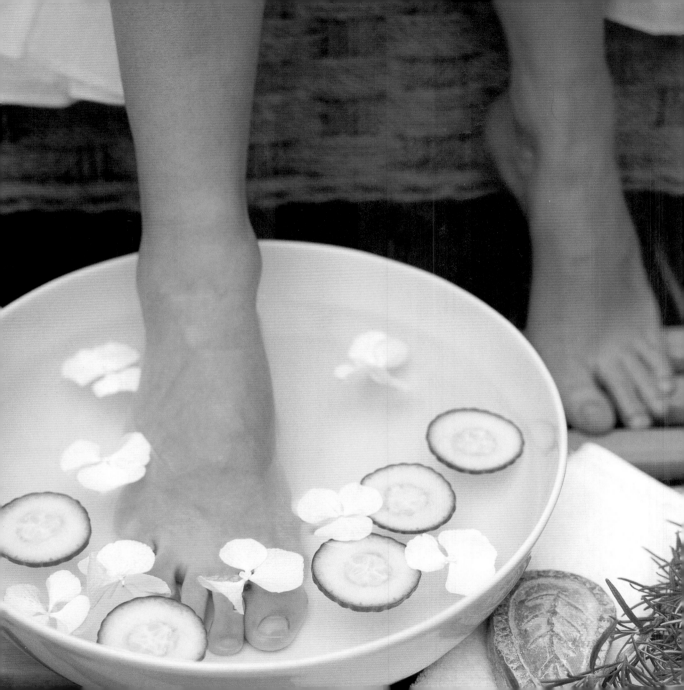

home treatments

Beyond doing pedicures, manicures and self-tanning at home, consider indulging in a few alternative beauty treatments that benefit not only the way you look, but also how you feel.

from spa to home

Bring the spa experience right into your home with deluxe beauty treatments to cocoon and pamper. Sometimes skin demands a little bit extra, especially in times of stress, so look to a skin-saving solution with a freshly made mask. After a soothing facial steam (add lavender or chamomile oils), apply the following:

HEAVENLY HONEY FACE MASK

A superlative moisturising mask for plump, soft skin.

2 tsps honey

2 tsps aloe vera gel

1 vitamin E capsule

Mix together the honey and aloe vera gel. Snip open the vitamin E capsule and squeeze in. Mix together, then apply to a freshly cleansed face. Leave for 10 minutes and rinse off.

THE ULTIMATE HAND AND FOOT TREAT

This mask will soften even the roughest of skin. You can apply it to elbows and knees, too.

1 avocado, finely mashed

1 egg yolk

1 tsp honey

3 tsps oat bran

5 drops evening primrose oil

Mix all the ingredients together, blending well, and gently massage onto hands and feet. Leave for 10 minutes and rinse.

BODY GLOW BLEND

A bespoke scrub is a luxury spa speciality.

1 cup fine sea salt

1 cup jojoba oil

2 drops eucalyptus essential oil

Mix all the ingredients together in a bowl. Dampen skin under the shower, then take a handful of the salt and oil mixture and massage into your skin. Rinse away with warm water.

LIP SLICK-ON

A super-kissable lip balm for pure seduction!

2 tsps beeswax

2 tsps almond oil

Place a water-filled saucepan over the heat. Put beewax into a bowl and place on saucepan. Mix the oil into the melted wax. Leave to cool in a small pot.

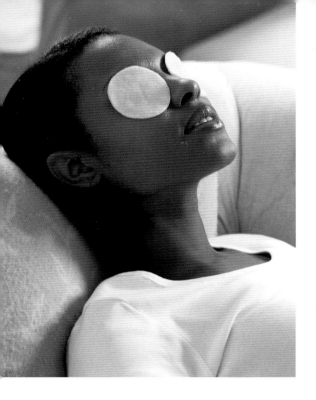

☆ *Give yourself a good foot rub and channel your solar plexus. You'll find it just below the ball of the foot. Press with your thumb to help balance the nervous system.*

☆ *For bright-eyed appeal, soak two cottonwool pads in lukewarm green tea and then place over the eyes. Green tea is a natural anti-inflammatory and will help decongest the eye area.*

☆ *Drink lots of water after any treatments, as your body has been detoxing.*

STAR SPA TIPS

• The night before your wedding, apply a lifting and firming mask to your neck and chest area, to give a natural uplift.

• Before beginning a treatment, put a towelling robe on a radiator. Post-treatment, you can cocoon up in it.

• Take time out to massage in moisture. A firm stroking technique will stimulate the lymphatic system, which carries toxins and waste from your cells.

• In preparation for being on your feet all day, strengthen your arches by running them slowly over a rolling pin.

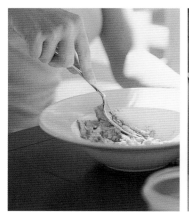

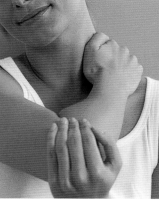

heading off pre-wedding stress

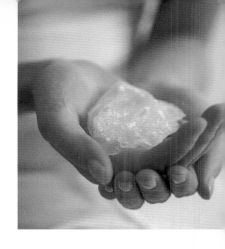

Organising a wedding can be chaotic, so soothe your senses, relax your mind and find an escape with these tension-melting ideas to free your mind.

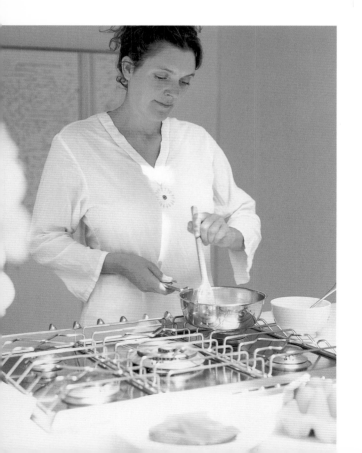

EAT YOURSELF CALM Brown rice, sweet potatoes and pasta all boast serotonin – a relaxing chemical that calms your mood. Munch bananas too. They contain vitamin B6, which builds serotonin levels. If you're on the pill, you could be depleting your body of this vitamin.

SPINAL SUSPENSION This is a stress-relieving pose that rids stress from the body. Find space and hang down like a rag doll over your thighs. Keep your knees soft. This pose is great for releasing trapped tension from the hips, shoulders and neck, and bringing a fresh supply of oxygen-rich blood to the brain for improved memory and concentration.

REACH A QUIET HIGH Deep breathing has been scientifically proven to lower blood pressure. Next time a situation is stressing you out, breathe out the stress. Sit with your back straight and chest relaxed. Breathe in deeply and fill your lungs as deep as you can. Release it

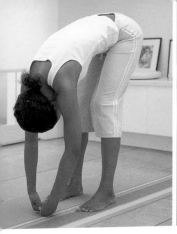
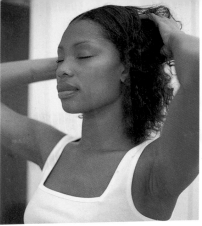
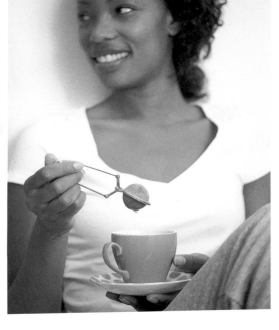

through your mouth, silently repeating 'Calm tummy, calm tummy'. Repeat three times until tranquil.

COLOUR YOURSELF CALM Wear green. In terms of colour therapy, it's the colour of new beginnings, has a positive effect on the immune system and promotes harmony in the body.

DON'T SAY A WORD! Give up talking. Although it may sound antisocial, 'verbal fasting' is becoming a way to find a moment of respite. Disciplining yourself to remain silent for a certain period is a great way to cleanse your mind, ground yourself and prioritise your thoughts.

NO NEWS IS GOOD NEWS If you wake up feeling tense, avoid listening to the news. People under stress internalize bad news, so hearing about famine or war may exacerbate any worries you already have. Put on some relaxing, slow-tempo music instead.

FROM FRAZZLED TO RELAXED

☆ *Use the 24-hour rule and sleep on big decisions. It doesn't matter who is hassling you for answers – wait a day, and then reply.*

☆ *Sip lemon balm tea. It increases feelings of serenity.*

☆ *Dip into some hubby-to-be! Touch slows the output of the stress hormone cortisol while giving a surge of the feel-good brain chemicals.*

☆ *Appeal to your sense of smell. According to aromachology - the study of how fragrance affects moods – rose is perceived as relaxing. Spritz a rose-filled fragrance to restore a sense of peace.*

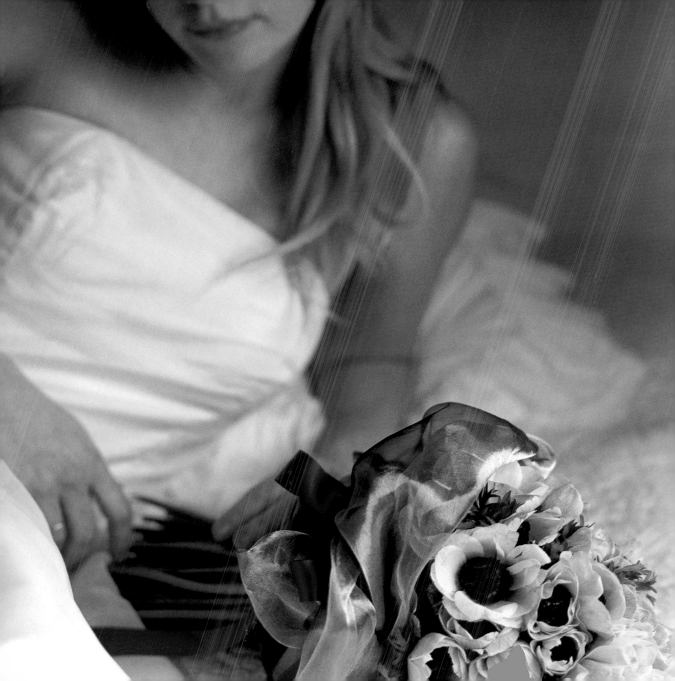

perfect bride

You've got the perfect man... Now all you want is to be the perfect-looking bride. With insider secrets on choosing the right gown, the low-down on figure-enhancing lingerie and clever tips for hair and make-up, it's never been so easy to look beautiful all day long!

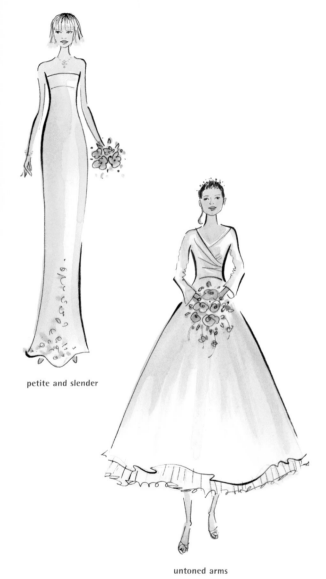

petite and slender

untoned arms

choosing your bridal-gown style

Your wedding dress has a lot to live up to, as guests will be buzzing with excitement to see it. The perfect dress will accentuate your good points and minimize any flaws. It will also give you confidence, as well as being comfortable to wear and utterly gorgeous!

PETITE AND SLENDER Empire-line dresses have a seam just below the bust and fall away to the floor. It's a style that suits slim and smaller-busted women. A column dress with a high neck is a style that can be pulled off by those blessed with a slight figure. Steer clear of ball gowns, which can swamp a petite figure.

UNTONED ARMS If you feel self-conscious of your arms, don't show them. Either opt for a dress with full sleeves, or choose a sleeveless dress, but cover your arms with a pretty jacket, shrug or wrap for a hint of movie-star glamour.

HOURGLASS FIGURE Consider a halter-neck gown, which gives the illusion of extending the shoulder line

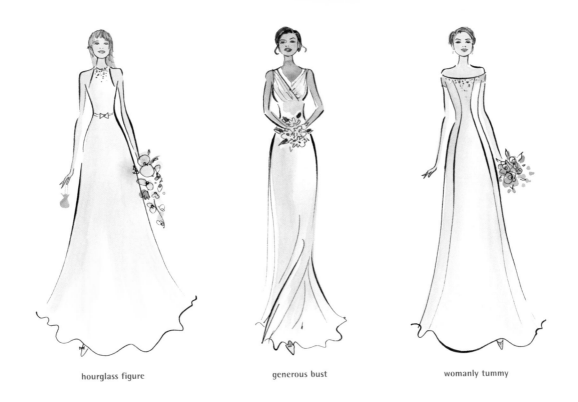

hourglass figure   generous bust   womanly tummy

and balancing out the lower body. A two piece works well if your bust is smaller than your hips. A bodice married with a ballerina-style skirt gives the figure a better proportion. Avoid straight or bias-cut designs, which magnify the hips and bottom.

GENEROUS BUST A strapless gown can look bewitching on a curvy figure, but you will need some extra support in the bust area (see undercover secrets, pages 44—45). A V-shaped or scooped neckline (not too plunging) is also flattering. Avoid high necklines, which make breasts appear larger.

WOMANLY TUMMY An A-line gown is perfect. This style flares out from the waist and hides a multitude of sins! Many A-line dresses have vertical seams running from the top of the dress to the bottom, so there are no seams across the dress at the tummy area. Leave the beading to the upper part of your dress. Avoid bows or sashes around the waist, as they will only add bulk.

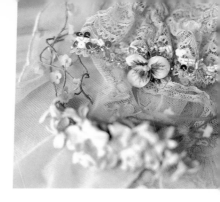

undercover secrets

Lingerie should be so much more than an afterthought. The right underwear is the hidden support you need to make your figure look better and your dress look amazing. Just as you should choose a dress to flatter your shape, so you should choose underwear to suit the style of your dress – think of it as a fail-safe foundation. Buy your wedding-day lingerie before you start your dress fittings, as it may alter your shape slightly.

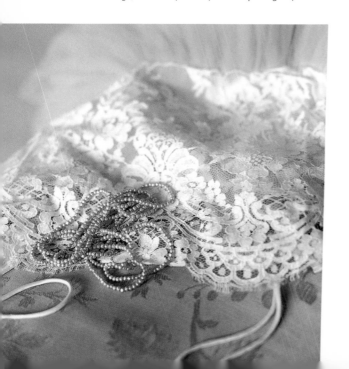

FIGURE-SKIMMING SILHOUETTE First off, check the colour of your bra under the dress – it should be completely invisible. Consider seamfree underwear, which makes for super-smooth foundations.

BOLD AND LOW-BACKED Unless you're very small breasted, don't think you won't need support for a strapless solution. Go for an adhesive bra. Shop around for different styles to suit your dress. The support is less than that of a regular bra, but they will hold the breasts in place, provide coverage, and give some shape.

SWEET AND STRAPLESS Strapless bras are ideal for strappy or low-cut dresses. Why not sew your bra into the dress? It will give you extra support and ensure the dress doesn't slide down and cause a revealing moment!

GENEROUS FIGURE Tackle trouble spots with control underwear, otherwise known as shapewear. Hold-you-in basques, pants and bras are an easy route to a cinched-in waist, higher bottom or flatter tummy.

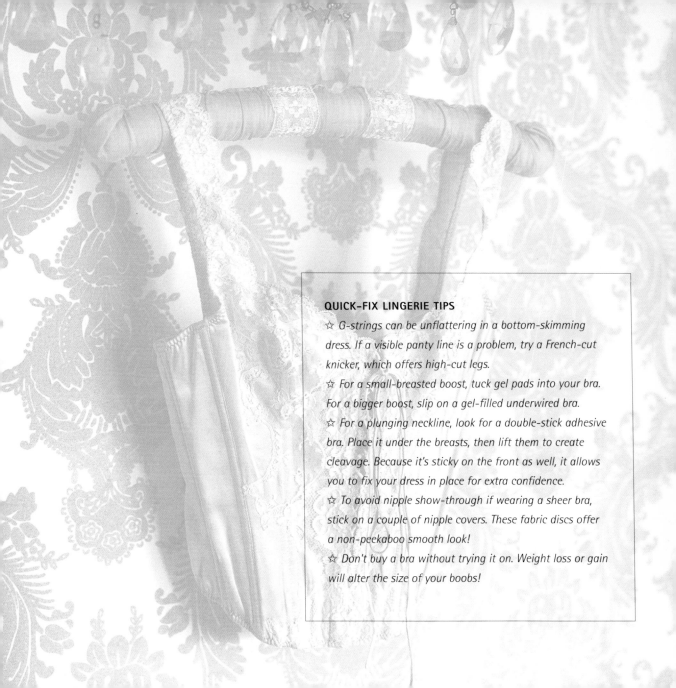

QUICK–FIX LINGERIE TIPS

☆ G-strings can be unflattering in a bottom-skimming dress. If a visible panty line is a problem, try a French-cut knicker, which offers high-cut legs.

☆ For a small-breasted boost, tuck gel pads into your bra. For a bigger boost, slip on a gel-filled underwired bra.

☆ For a plunging neckline, look for a double-stick adhesive bra. Place it under the breasts, then lift them to create cleavage. Because it's sticky on the front as well, it allows you to fix your dress in place for extra confidence.

☆ To avoid nipple show-through if wearing a sheer bra, stick on a couple of nipple covers. These fabric discs offer a non-peekaboo smooth look!

☆ Don't buy a bra without trying it on. Weight loss or gain will alter the size of your boobs!

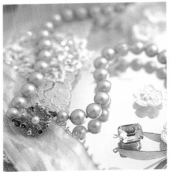
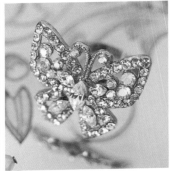
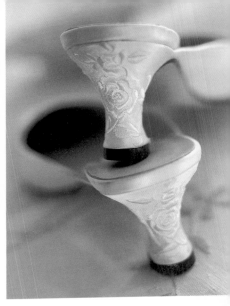

luxury bits and pieces

Just like the dress, your wedding accessories should be planned and thought out with care. Accessorising with style adds glamour and panache to your whole look.

JEWELLERY It may be tempting to wear Grandma's diamond earrings, the bracelet your mother bought you and a pendant your beau gave you, but if you don't want to look like a fairground attraction, opt just for a couple of pieces. Harmonize any stones found in your dress or headpiece with those in the jewels you choose. Pearls will complement beading, whereas diamonds go well with sequins or crystals. Let your hairstyle and headpiece dictate the earrings. Bejewelled drop earrings look great with an upswept do, while studs won't steal the fanfare from a decorative headpiece.

HEADDRESS The headpiece you choose will depend on whether your hair is long or short or whether you are wearing it up or down. Like your jewellery, your style of headpiece will reflect your personality – you can keep it low-key or go for something theatrical. Once only seen on the heads of society brides, tiaras are now worn by modern brides with great aplomb. Decorative headbands in the fabric of your dress can look great, as can jewelled combs for shoulder-length hair. Feathers and flowers can be used either in a headdress or woven into the hair.

GLOVES AND SHRUGS For gloves, match the colour to your wedding dress, and pair simple gloves with decorative dresses, or more elaborate gloves with a simple gown. As for length, wear a glove that ends just below or above the elbow with a short-sleeved dress, an 'opera' glove (to just below the armpit) with a strapless gown, and wrist-length gloves with a long-sleeved dress. Remove gloves just before the ceremony, wear them for formal photographs and take them off when eating! Ask your dressmaker about cover-ups. A long tailored coat, bolero, pashmina or a shrug are all good choices.

SHOES Wedding shoes need to look elegant as well as be comfortable. The height of your shoes is important. If you're not relaxed in high heels, your wedding is not the best time to wear them! Consider lower kitten heels or a ballet slipper, which look very pretty with a ballerina-length gown. Don't feel restricted to 'wedding' shoes, either — go beyond bridal, and shop around.

FRAGRANCE Fragrance has a powerful effect on memory, so you want to wear a scent that will make your heart lift whenever you smell it again. If you're thinking about wearing a different 'wedding' scent, leave yourself time to sniff out something new. Don't forget to ask your partner if he likes your choice! Weddings are full of emotions and the body heat that's generated will intensify any fragrance, so bear that in mind before wearing a potent scent. Consider the seasons, too. A fresh floral scent is perfect in spring and summer, whereas a heavy oriental scent would be more suitable in autumn or winter.

ACCESSORY TIPS
- If you choose flowers for your hair, talk to your florist about the best types to use. You need robust blooms rather than ones that wilt quickly.
- If you have a hand-tied bouquet, ask the florist to wind the ribbon all the way down the stems. You don't want them snagging your dress or gloves.
- Try on wedding shoes at the end of the day, when your feet are at their largest.
- Make sure there's a large umbrella in the wedding car, just in case it rains.

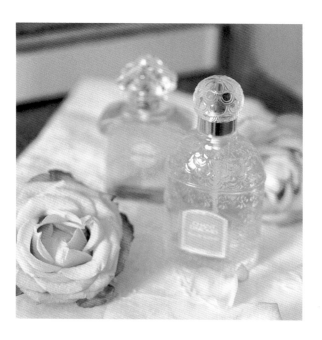

a head-turning affair

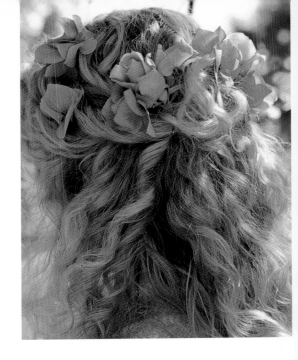

Now the condition of your hair is enhanced with good nutrition, and the texture and shine improved with good products, it's time to find the perfect hairstyle.

BEFRIEND YOUR STYLIST Three months before the wedding is a good time to start discussing ideas with your stylist. Take along pictures of looks you like, so they can advise on what style will suit your face shape. If you want your stylist to do your hair on your wedding day, book them early and make sure they are totally happy with the date. There's nothing worse than having a stylist cancel at the last minute.

THE TRIAL RUN Once you have booked your stylist and chosen your headpiece, make an appointment with your stylist around two weeks before your wedding day, to try out the various looks. Let them know the style of your dress, as it will dictate how you wear your hair.

A STYLE TO SUIT YOU Whether you want to sweep your hair up into a chignon, wear it in a beehive or dress in a stylish knot, your face shape is an important factor. There are a few general rules on choosing a style to flatter your face.

LONG FACE
• Hair pulled back from the face will only elongate the face further. It's flattering to have a few wispy strands tumbling down from the crown and in front of the ears.
• Avoid styles that sit on top of the head. Instead, opt for buns or knots on the back of the head, as this will balance out your features.
• If you're wearing your hair down, do not part in the middle. Go for a side parting.

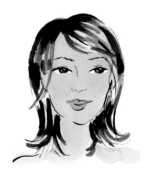

long face

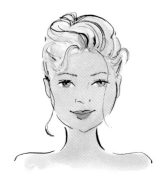

round face

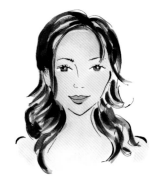

heart shape face

ROUND FACE

• Longer hair strands falling onto and around the face give the illusion that your face is longer and slimmer.

• Loose curls piled on top of the head or a relaxed up-do will give the effect of a more shapely face. They will also add extra height for anyone wanting to appear taller.

HEART SHAPE

• Inject some fullness into the bottom half of your face with falling tendrils and waves that finish at the chin. This will also make a large forehead seem less broad.

GOING TO GREAT LENGTHS Of course, the length of your hair will have some influence when it comes to choosing the right style. There's no point hankering after a style if your hair just isn't long enough!

LONG HAIR There are endless ways to wear long hair. You can pile it up into a classic chignon or a chic beehive, making a great base for your chosen headpiece.

MEDIUM-LENGTH HAIR If you want to put your hair up but are worried there's not enough length, ask your stylist about a hair sponge. These are doughnut-shaped pieces of sponge that come in colours to match your hair shade. They're placed on the crown, and hair is pinned around them. This tricks the eye into thinking you actually have more hair than you have. Low ponytails at the nape of the neck can also look stylish.

SHORT HAIR Short hair relies on a good cut. From then on, either keep your style simple or dress it up. Try a diamanté headband, a tiara or tiny crystal hairclips.

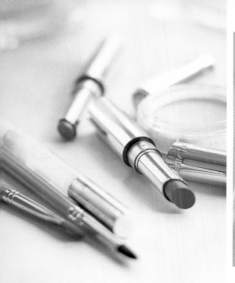

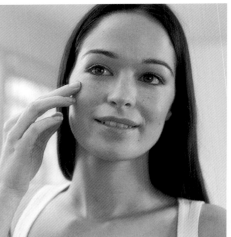

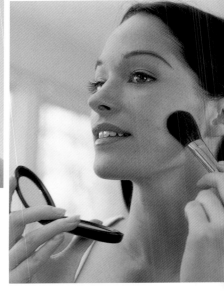

lovely make-up

On your wedding day, subtly applied make-up is essential and will help bring out the star in you.

EXPERT HELP The secret to great make-up is keeping it simple, along with a little know-how on what products to choose and how to use them. This is where a professional make-up artist comes into their own. If you are having your make-up applied professionally on the day, meet up a few weeks beforehand to discuss your look, and have a trial run before the big day. When looking for a make-up artist, word of mouth is your best option. If no one offers up names, ask around.

DO-IT-YOURSELF If you are doing your own make-up, head for your nearest department store and enquire at leading cosmetic counters about a bridal consultation. You'll be shown some professional techniques, as well as hues to suit your skintone. This should make you more confident about applying your make-up on the day.

FLAWLESS COMPLEXION Apply a primer before applying foundation. They form an invisible barrier between your skin and make-up, so foundation stays put. You don't want a heavy-looking base, so keep it light, choosing a foundation that covers any blemishes

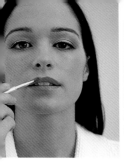
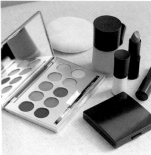

but also allows the skin to breathe. Blend foundation outwards and upwards from your nose. Cover any blemishes with a concealer that matches your skintone. Finish with a light dusting of translucent powder.

PRETTY CHEEKS A flush of colour on the cheeks makes for a pretty and youthful look. Blend a cream blush from your cheekbones up to your temples. Swirl over a dusting of powder blush to help the blush last all day.

INCREDIBLE EYES Prep the eyelids with eyeshadow primer or face powder to help colour stay put. Play it safe by brushing just one shade over the lid, from lashes to socket. Resist the temptation to go for brightly coloured hues. If you want to use something more exciting than taupe – sparkly gold powder, perhaps – apply the eyeshadow with a dampened brush. This makes for a less glittery and more shimmery feel. Run an eye pencil close to the roots of your upper lashes, then smudge the outer corners. Curl your eyelashes and apply two coats of waterproof mascara.

LUSCIOUS LIPS Kissing, eating and sipping champagne can take its toll on your lipstick, so either wear a long-lasting formula, or line and fill the mouth with a neutral lip pencil for extra staying power. Bear in mind shades close to your own lip colour are low-maintenance and can be reapplied quickly. A dramatic red can look striking but will need frequent reapplying.

MAKE-UP TRICKS AND TIPS

☆ *Bring a little sparkle to arms and shoulders by mixing a tiny bit of pearlised face powder into your body lotion.*

☆ *If you're having a facial, make sure it's at least a week prior to the wedding. Facials can be detoxing on the skin, resulting in blemishes.*

☆ *A silvery white shadow brushed across the eyes makes the whites of the eyes look even whiter and is a fabulous look for blondes and baby-blue eyes.*

☆ *Face shine is your number one enemy in pictures. Make sure you have a compact of ultra-light powder in your bag so you can give yourself a fine dusting before smiling for the camera.*

☆ *Avoid lip gloss if you're wearing a veil – it will stick to your lips. Instead, use a slick of petroleum jelly.*

do's and don't's before your wedding day

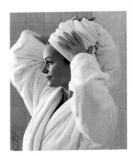
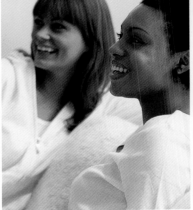

THE NIGHT BEFORE

• Don't drink large amounts of alcohol. It will dehydrate you, encourage a hangover, and won't make you look or feel good on the day.

• Do spend time with people who relax you.

• Don't eat gas-causing foods such as beans, broccoli and cauliflower. They can all cause bloating and wind.

• Do check buttons and zips on your gown. And hang it out of harm's way!

• Don't take sleeping pills. You'll feel groggy the next morning. Go for a herbal tea or warm milk instead.

• Do get some beauty sleep. A few drops of lavender essential oil on your pillow equals restful sleep. If possible, sleep on your back. It lessens the risk of crease lines on your face and décolletage.

• Do make a timetable for getting ready, and stick to it!

• Don't expect everything to run smoothly. Add in an extra hour (set your alarm) in case of any last-minute glitches, such as a broken nail.

• Do wish your partner luck before bedtime. It's his big day tomorrow too, and he's sure to be feeling nervous!

THE BIG DAY

• Do run an early bath and enjoy time on your own.

• Don't get too friendly with a champagne breakfast. You don't want to be burping or slurring your vowels!

• Do soak two cotton pads in lukewarm green tea and place them on puffy eyes for 10 minutes. A natural anti-inflammatory, the tea will decongest the area.

• Don't pick up your bouquet if pollen hasn't been removed from the stamens. It may stain your dress.

• Do compliment your bridesmaids, maid of honour and mother on how lovely they look.

• Don't panic about creases in your veil. Simply use your hairdryer on a medium setting to remove the wrinkles.

• Do keep your sense of humour and remember that this day is about love and celebration. Relax, smile and enjoy!

• Don't be embarrassed about shedding a tear or two.

• Do look to a holistic fix to stay calm. Drop Bach's Rescue Remedy onto your tongue before you enter the church – it's the hip way to calm nerves.

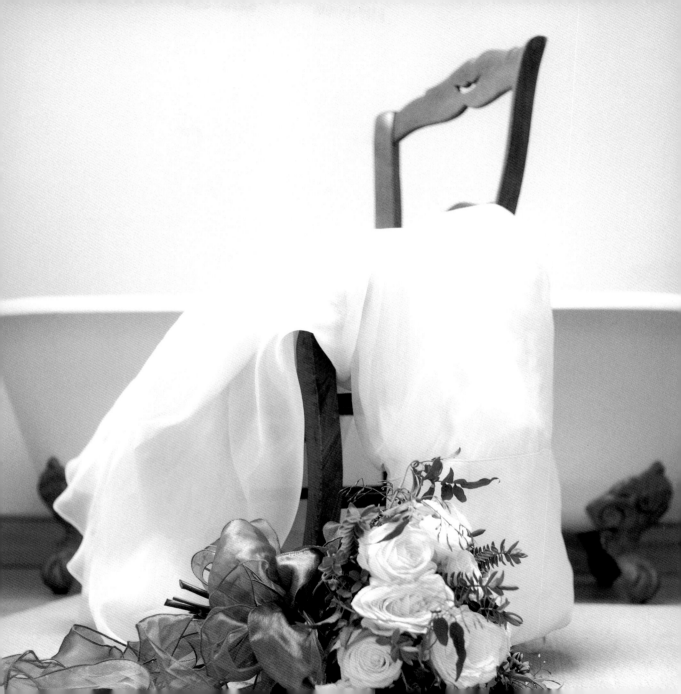

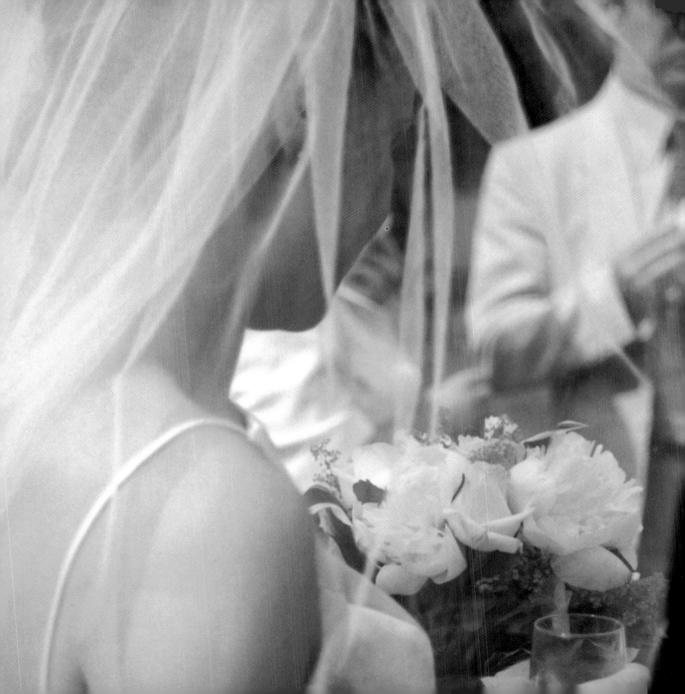

the big day

Months of precise planning have finally come to fruition, and it's your wedding day! Take deep, meditative breaths to soothe any last-minute nerves and follow a few essential prep steps to ensure your big day goes smoothly.

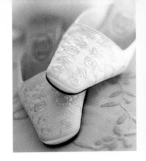

essential prep steps

THE BASICS Apply deodorant and body lotions as early as possible, so they have time to sink into your skin. You do not want to be a bride who reveals cakey white armpits, so use a stainless roll-on deodorant. Eat a decent breakfast and make sure you have more than just a quick coffee. There's nothing worse than the sound of

a rumbling tummy during the ceremony, or feeling faint or light-headed through hunger! Oats have a calming effect, so eat some porridge, oatcakes or flapjacks. Put on some soothing, relaxing music, and, if your bridesmaids or mother are getting ready with you, don't be afraid to make them responsible for minor jobs that will help you keep organized.

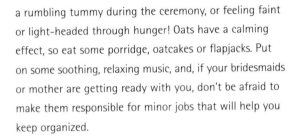

HAIR AND MAKE-UP Dress in comfortable clothes while you're having your hair and make-up done. Make sure they're easy to remove and don't have to go over your head – the last thing you want to do is mess up your hair! Whether you're doing your make-up yourself or having a professional team, enjoy the pampering. If you are doing your own make-up, leave plenty of time. If your headdress has pearls in it, remember to spray your hair before fixing it in place (hairspray ruins pearls).

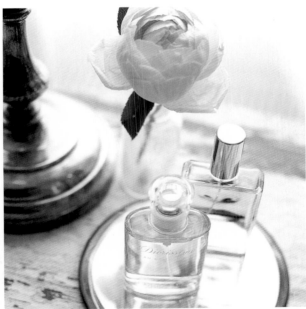

CLEVER DRESSING If your dress is low-backed or strapless, do not wear a bra on the morning of the wedding, as it can cause skin marks that take hours to fade. When it's time to get dressed, slip on your underwear, bra, stockings, petticoat and garter. Now step into your dress. Allow 15 minutes to slowly fasten and adjust the dress. Zip and button it up little by little to avoid a broken zipper or pulled-off buttons. A long gown needs static protection, so spray a static guard generously. This makes sure the only thing that clings to you closely is your groom! Put on your shoes, first having scored the soles with a knife or scuffed them with a nail file so they are not slippery. Swap your engagement ring to your right hand and put on the rest of your jewellery. When you move, be sure to hold a long dress up gently. Clutching it in a sweaty palm will only cause wrinkles.

BAGS OF STYLE You only need somewhere to slip a lipstick and compact, so think lightweight, delicate and small when it comes to bags. When choosing a bag, make sure it complements the colour and the fabric of your dress. Remember that clutch bags need to be carried in your hands, while a small handbag can dangle from the wrist, leaving hands free to meet and greet guests.

BRIDAL EMERGENCY KIT

Be prepared! Put together an emergency kit and give to your maid of honour or a bridesmaid. Include a small sewing kit, tissues, mints, stockings, the nail polish you are wearing (nothing looks worse than a chipped nail), hairbrush, headache tablets, eye drops and baby powder (useful for any spills on the dress).

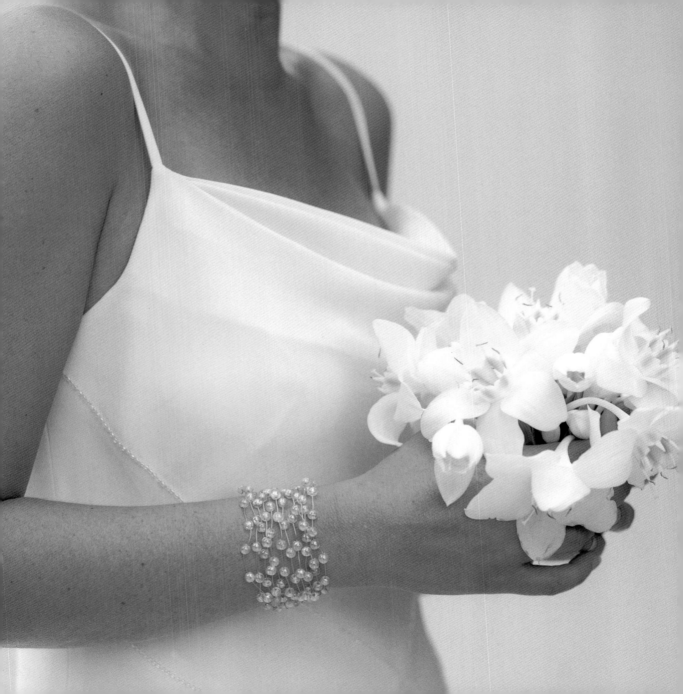

making your entrance

Eye-catching gems and a stunning wedding dress certainly get you noticed, but it's the small details that make for a truly beautiful bride.

POSTURE PERFECT Standing tall tells the world (and the congregation) that you feel great about yourself. A few simple techniques are all it takes to look instantly taller and leaner. Straighten your back, drop your shoulders, pull in your stomach and try to hold this position when walking, standing and sitting. Control your arms and keep them parallel to the body as much as possible. Finally, lengthen your neck and tilt your chin upwards for an air of relaxed confidence.

EXITING A CAR GRACEFULLY It's a pretty simple technique. Before the door is opened, straighten your dress and swivel your knees towards the door. When the door is open, swing both legs out at the same time and stand up. The biggest mistake is sticking one leg out, then the other. That's when you risk letting more than your garter show! If you are wearing a wrap, put it on after you exit the car. Don't get out clutching everything; otherwise, you'll look like a bag lady!

GLIDE, DON'T STRIDE Heels add inches to your height. Just make sure you glide in them for maximum effect. The secret to an elegant walk lies in overlapping your feet rather than walking with them side by side. This makes for a clomping walk rather than a graceful effect. Shorten your steps and step with your heel first, then let the sole follow quickly and smoothly. Walk with your toes pointing straight ahead and keep your legs straight, close and parallel. When it comes to wedding shoes, avoid mules. They're very hard to keep on and walk in elegantly for a long period of time.

LOOKING GOOD IN PHOTOGRAPHS There are rules to follow for giving a good picture. First, practise your pose. Turn your body slightly to the side so you aren't facing the camera straight on, place one foot in front of the other, move your chest and neck forwards and stick your bottom out slightly. This will elongate and angle your body wonderfully. To avoid a double chin, lift your head up slightly and angle it to the side to define your bone structure. If you find yourself squinting move out of the sun, and if you have amalgam fillings don't throw your head back and laugh!

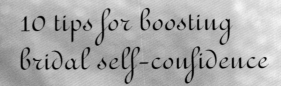

10 tips for boosting bridal self-confidence

You look fabulous – now you want to feel it! For sky-high confidence, lighten your emotional load and look to ways of boosting your self-esteem.

1 If feeling nervous, focus on love. It sounds corny, but when you think of someone you really love – your soon-to-be-husband – you can't really experience nerves and love at the same time.

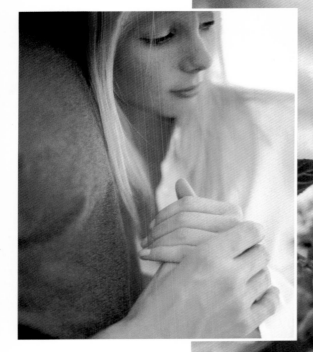

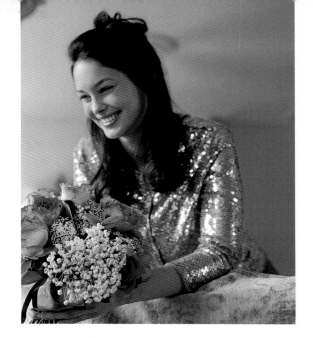

2 Maintain good eye contact when you're exchanging vows with your partner. It helps you feel strong, lays nerves to rest, and shows that you feel confident and believe in what you're saying.

3 Remember to touch your partner. With all the attention and people vying for your company, it can be easy to lose sight – as well as touch – of each other. Take time to hold hands and give each other little kisses when the camera and eyes are off you. Not only does touch release feel-good chemicals, it revitalizes you too.

4 If you feel tension building up, shake your arms and legs loosely for a few minutes. The physical movement releases stress, and the spontaneity is freeing.

5 Think yourself fabulous... because you are! Positive thinking can help your mind get to where you want it to be. Shake off any last-minute doubts and stresses by saying to yourself 'I look gorgeous!'

6 Give compliments graciously throughout the day. There is no greater confidence than making someone else feel great about themselves, too.

7 Speak up and keep your voice strong and clear. Your voice reveals your emotions, so a joyful and confident tone will say it all.

8 Be friends with everyone at the reception. There's often an undercurrent of family tension at large gatherings, so choose to ignore it and delight in the fact that everybody is celebrating for you. This action will make your day even more special.

9 Have fun. It's a party! The more laid-back and care-free you are, the more confident you become.

10 Remind yourself you're getting a loving partner for life. What could be a bigger confidence booster?

sources

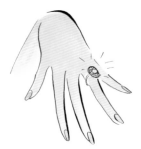

NUTRITION AND FITNESS

The Nutrition Coach
0845 0502 442
www.thenutritioncoach.co.uk
Clinical nutritionists that develop
do-able tailor-made programmes
and who believe on being on call
via telephone and email. Acne,
brittle nails, skin conditions and
anxiety are all areas they can
help with through nutrition.

Sarah Maxwell Fitness &
Lifestyle Consultancy
020 8542 3754
www.sarahmaxwell.co.uk
A personal trainer who has
shaped up many a bride-to-be
and who believes in all kinds of
disciplines, including Pilates,
yoga, weight training and
cardiovascular development.

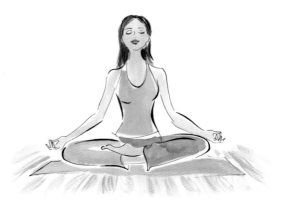

SKINCARE

The Alternative Centre
The White House
Roxby Place
London SW6 1RS
020 7381 2298
Specialists in natural
dermatology. Focus on clearing
troubled skin conditions (such as
acne and psoriasis) naturally,

Leonard Drake Skincare
Centres
8 Lancer Street
Kensington Church Street
London W8 4EH
020 7937 7060
and
The Cloisters Mall
Kingston-upon-Thames
Surrey KT1 1RS
020 8541 0999
Customized facials using
Dermalogica products and Face
Mapping skin analysis.

EYEBROWS

The Blink Bar
Fenwicks
New Bond Street
London W1A 3BS
020 7629 9161
A walk-in eyebrow-shaping
service using threading.

HAIR AND MAKE-UP

Benefit
0901 11300001
www.benefitcosmetics.com
Create perfect make-up with
their 'Fake it' range – magical
products that conceal and
enhance.

Bobbi Brown Studio
0870 034 2566
Complimentary make-up lessons
with professional make-up
artists. During the half-hour
session, you will receive a
personalized look and learn tricks
of the trade. All the products
used are recorded on a face chart
that you can reference when
recreating your look at home.

Estée Lauder Bridal Beauty
0870 034 6822
Three consultations leading up to
and after the wedding cover
personalized skincare and expert
make-up advice.

Michaeljohn
25 Albemarle Street
London W1S 4HU
020 7629 6969
Offers face and body treatments

as well as hair and make-up. All
hairstylists and therapists will do
home visits.

The Perfect Marriage
www.theperfectmarriage.co.uk
Jo Lewis (top hairstylist) and Jo
Edwards (leading make-up artist)
will come to your home and
provide a totally bespoke service
based on the wedding look you
want to achieve.

Richard Ward Hair and
Metrospa
82 Duke of York Square
London SW3 4LY
020 7730 1222
www.richardward.co.uk
Specialist bridal stylists will
analyse your hair's capabilities
and discuss your bridal look. They
offer a bridal hair consultation
and trial and a bridal make-up
trial. Home visits are available on
quotation.

PAMPERING AND TANNING

Champneys Health Resorts
08703 300 300
www.champneys.com
A selection of packages to
beautify and relax you.

Fantasy Tan

020 8498 7266 for nearest salon

The Fantasy Tan Bridal Formula is specially designed for your wedding day. It is formulated not to rub off on clothing and is applied using a clear spray that adds a little sparkle. As the sparkle fades, you are left with a rich tan for your honeymoon.

Heaven@home

0871 200 1282

www.heavenathome.net

Bring the salon to your home for a pampering night. Their team offer beauty treatments and a range of alternative therapies.

The Janet Ginnings Hair & Beauty Salon

45 Curzon Street

London W1Y 7UQ

020 7499 1904

Janet's Indian Kitchen Body Conditioning Treatment uses goat's milk, oils and spice and leaves skin soft and revitalized.

St Tropez Tanning

0115 983 6363

The company that transformed the fake-tan market. Call the above number for information on stockists, salons and local therapists who make home visits.

Touch

020 7935 2205

www.londontouch.com

Brings holistic therapists and beauty specialists to your home. Choose from over 40 treatments, from massage to manicures.

FRAGRANCE

Jo Malone

23 Brook Street

London W1K 4HA

020 7491 9104

Fragrance Combining encourages you to combine two or more scents to create a fragrance that is completely your own.

WEDDING GOWNS

Basia Zarzycka

52 Sloane Square

London SW1V 8AX

020 7730 1660

www.basia-zarzycka.co.uk

A treasure trove of tiaras, wedding gowns and shoes.

Debenhams

www.debenhams.com

Designers at Debenhams consists of 20 different ready-to-wear bridal dresses, including J by Jasper Conran and PIIF by

Pearce Fionda, available in 24 stores nationwide. Also accessories.

Mirror Mirror

37 Park Road

London N8 8TE

020 8348 2113

Dresses for celebrities and the discerning bride-to-be.

Virgin Bride

35 King Street

Manchester M2 7AT

08700 600 436

Gowns, bridesmaids' dresses and bridal accessories.

The Wedding Shop at Liberty

210–220 Regent Street

London W1B 5AH

020 7734 1234

Liberty stock two designers, namely Vera Wang and Elie Saab who dress A-list celebrities for red-carpet appearances.

WEDDING SHOES

Emma Hope

33 Amwell Street

London EC1 1UR

020 7833 2367

White satin shoes with lattice, pleat and bow details and some matching bags.

BRIDAL UNDERWEAR

Agent Provocateur

6 Broadwick Street

London W1F 8HL

020 7439 0229

This saucy lingerie shop reveals

that brides indulge in classic lingerie for their wedding day, but prefer something a little naughtier for the honeymoon!

Rigby & Peller

22A Conduit Street

London W1S 2XT

020 7491 2200

An expert fitting service and extensive ranges of bras, knickers and corsets.

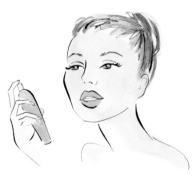

WEDDING PLANNER

Rebecca Hulme-Richardson

0115 979 5891

www.theweddingandpartyplanner.co.uk

Rebecca can advise on all aspects of your wedding, including hair and make-up, and offer fashion guidance, too.

USEFUL WEBSITES

www.confetti.co.uk

www.theukweddingsshows.co.uk

www.guidesforbrides.co.uk

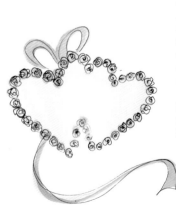

picture credits

Key: a=above, b=below, r=right, l=left, c=centre.
All illustrations by Robyn Neilb. All photographs by Winfried Heinze, unless otherwise stated.

Daniel Farmer: pages 19a, 24, 37al, 37br, 50c, 50r, 51l, 51c, 52 both. Claire Richardson: endpapers, pages 28, 34, 44, 45, 46l, 46c, 47, 56l. Dan Duchars: pages 5ar both, 23b, 26l, 27b, 29r, 38l, 50l, 54. Craig Fordham: pages 1, 2, 3, 5l, 7, 20, 30l, 40, 53, 60r, 61. Polly Wreford: pages 4, 31l, 38r, 46r, 56r, 57, 58, 60l. David Montgomery: pages 19b, 25, 29l, 33ar, 36, 39b, 59. Chris Everard: pages 8, 26r. Caroline Arber: page48. Nicki Dowey: page 22r. Andrew Wood: page 37ar.

acknowledgements

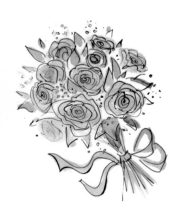

My own wedding was very small – but very beautiful. Whatever type of wedding you choose, a bride always needs to feel special, so I dedicate this book to my two friends Carolyn and Clive Boyland, who helped organise my wedding day and made me feel just that.

This book is a collection of insiders' tips passed onto me through interviewing many experts in the beauty and fashion industry. There are so many people I would like to thank, but special thanks must go to Michelle Marsh and Ariane Poole for their invaluable make-up tips, Wendy Carrig for her brilliant photographic insights, Janet Ginnings for her colonic cleanser recipe, Kate Cook for her advice on nutrition and Sarah Maxwell, a wonderful personal trainer, for her exercise tips.

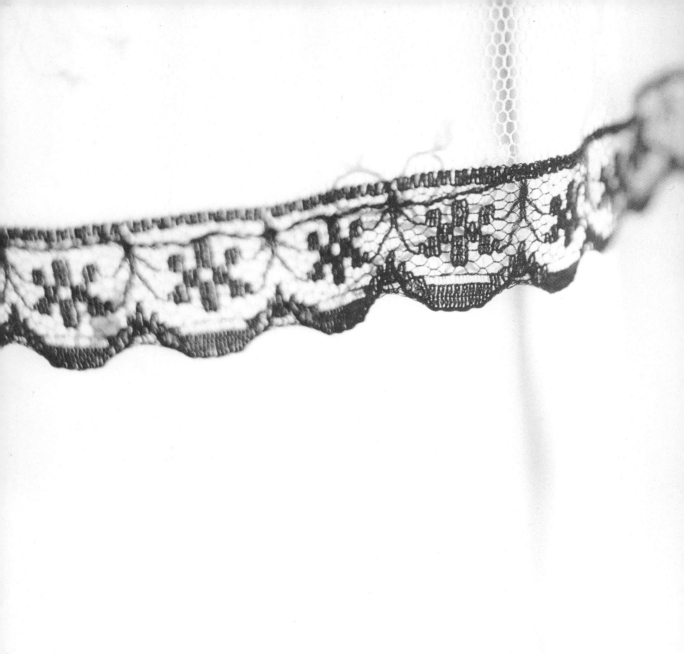